Genuine Nourishment
FOR PREGNANCY

Sound HABITS REAL Nourishment
FOR PREGNANCY

Forward

No matter what foods are practical for you daily, taking vitamins is an important component of making sure you get the nutrients you need. Vitamins make sure you are getting the nutrients you require daily for pregnancy for both you and your unborn child.

These ideas can be used to create a wholesome, well-balanced pregnancy diet. Everyone should have a nutritious diet that includes well-balanced meals and snacks, but pregnant women need to pay particular attention to this.

The health of expectant mothers and their unborn children depends on eating a balanced, nutritious diet. There are certain significant principles to bear in mind when eating during pregnancy, even though there isn't a one-size-fits-all approach to nutrition.

Table of content

- Beans
- Meats
- Berries
- Broccoli
- Chaddar
- Eggs
- Milk
- Squeeze Orange
- Pork Tenderloin
- Salmon
- Yam
- Entire grains
- Yogurt (plain, low-fat or sans fat)

Chapter 3: Solid Food During Pregnancy

- Food desire during Pregnancy
- Which Food varieties to eat and keep away from during pregnancy

Introduction:

Genuine Nourishment for Pregnancy

Growing a human is perhaps the most astounding thing our bodies achieve during its life. Maybe the coolest thing about it is, however, that tiny idea needs to go into the demonstration. After origination, a mother can approach her day-to-day existence giving little consideration to her developing embryo despite everything making a completely working human. Notwithstanding, an overall misguided judgment most ladies have is that whenever pregnancy has been laid out, there is minimal that should be possible to influence the development and strength of the child, that hereditarily talking the child will be what it is.

I'm here to let you know that this is just mostly obvious.

Chapter 1:

Genuine food varieties for sound Pregnancy and Kid

Genuine food sources

Indeed, people are wired to recreate accurately, in any event, when conditions are not ideal. In any case, the things that are inside a mother's control during pregnancy — diet, work out, rest propensities, stress, poison openness — can fundamentally affect the pregnancy and can leave long-lasting engravings on the child's wellbeing. Deficient nourishment during pregnancy can impede appropriate turn of events and lead to long-lasting metabolic changes that increment the gamble of infection. By zeroing in on legitimate supplement consumption during pregnancy, besides the fact that, a mother can make a superior outline for her developing child yet additionally her future grandkids and extraordinary grandkids.

So, why genuine food? Present day sustenance will in general detach and concentrate on single supplements rather than entire food sources. This is the reason a pre-birth is recommended to most pregnant ladies — it takes individual fixings and places it into one case. Food and supplements work synergistically, however, so why not take a gander at how food varieties cooperate related to the legitimate capability of the human body? Basically, red food is made with straightforward fixings that are as near to nature as could be expected and not handled such that it eliminates supplements. The following are a few central issues and ideas to search for while picking solid, genuine food sources.

Do we truly have to “eat for two” when pregnant? Actually, no, not, actually. By and large caloric admission just increments barely so ponder eating for 1.1. What is it that increments is the requirement for vitamin A, folate, vitamin B12, choline, iron, and iodine.

Carbs are the main thing that raise your glucose. Focus on carbs that are supplement thick and falling short on the glycemic file to assist with forestalling a spike in glucose and pointless weight gain.

Protein is the structure blocks of human existence! Each cell contains protein and is fundamental for new cell development, both for mother and child.

A body's requirement for fat-solvent nutrients goes up during pregnancy. A child's cerebrum is 60% fat, and that fat requirements come from some place.

Water is fundamental for keeping up with a great course, which carries supplements to children and eliminates byproducts. Hold back nothing day.

As a lady expands their water admission, electrolyte (counting salt) utilization should increment too. Electrolytes are important for cell and body capability, and low salt admission can deteriorate glucose and insulin opposition.

About the subject of eating "genuine food" during pregnancy

There are sure food sources that give fundamental nutrients and supplements to both mother and child. Recorded underneath, you will find a rundown of entire food decisions that any expecting mother ought to add to their eating routine. These are food varieties that form a sound child!

Eggs:

high in protein and contain a lot of choline, which is required for fetal mental health and deep-rooted memory upgrade. Pick eggs from field raised chickens for the greatest protein and fat substance.

Liver:

frequently depicted as nature's multivitamin, liver is plentiful in pretty much every nutrient and mineral that advanced nourishment has distinguished up to this point. It is the single most extravagant wellspring of iron, and furthermore contains folate, vitamin B12 and vitamin A. Look for liver from sound, field raised creatures.

Bone Stock:

the bone, skin, and connective tissues of creatures are plentiful in protein, collagen, gelatin, glycine, and minerals. When stewed, it makes an electrolyte drink like Gatorade.

Mixed Greens: dietary forces to be reckoned with that are moved in nutrients, minerals, and cancer prevention agents. They are the most plentiful wellspring of folate. Every one of the supplements in vegetables are fat-solvent, meaning they are best assimilated when consumed with sound fat.

Salmon and Greasy Fish:

Fish utilization in pregnancy is straightforwardly corresponded to higher youth level of intelligence and relational abilities. Be careful to keep away from ruler mackerel, tile fish and shark to keep away from elevated degrees of mercury; in any case, fish additionally contain selenium which ties with mercury and keeps it from applying its harmful impacts.

Full-Fat and Matured Dairy Items:

A critical wellspring of K2, which isn't broadly accessible in our eating regimens. This nutrient is fundamental for development of the fetal skeleton, and keeping up with the mother's skeletal bone thickness. It additionally assists with expanding insulin responsiveness, assisting with keeping up with ordinary glucose through pregnancy.

So, that's it. Eat genuine, entire food to assist with supporting a sound child and put yourself in a position for a brilliant pregnancy.

Eating Right When Pregnant

Great sustenance during pregnancy, and enough of it, is vital for your child to develop and create. You ought to consume around 300 additional calories each day (an additional 600 every day assuming you're conveying twins)than you did before you became pregnant.

Although queasiness and heaving during the initial not many long periods of pregnancy can make this troublesome, attempt to eat an even eating regimen and take pre-birth nutrients. Here are a few proposals to keep you and your child solid.

Objectives for Good dieting When Pregnant

Eat various food varieties to get every one of the supplements you really want. Suggested day-to-day servings incorporate 6-11 servings of breads and grains, two to four servings of natural product, at least four servings of vegetables, four servings of dairy items, and three servings of protein sources (meat, poultry, fish, eggs, or nuts). Consume fats and desserts sparingly.

Pick food sources high in fiber that are advanced, for example, entire grain breads, oats, beans, pasta and rice, as well as products of the soil. Although it's ideal to get your fiber from food varieties, taking a fiber supplement can assist you with getting the important sum. Models incorporate psyllium and methyl cellulose. Chat with your PCP before beginning any enhancements. If you take a fiber supplement, increment the sum you take gradually. This can assist with forestalling gas and squeezing. It's likewise vital to drink an adequate number of fluids when you increment your fiber consumption.

Protein drives blood creation, particularly when it has iron that your body effectively retains, as from red meats, chicken, and shellfish. Your blood volume increases during pregnancy to supply your child's blood as well. Choose sound proteins that aren't high in fat, similar to incline meats, fish, poultry, tofu and other soy items, beans, nuts, and egg whites.

You and your children need a few fats to remain sound. Simply make sure to pick the sound, unsaturated kind like vegetable oils, olive oil, and nuts.

Ensure you are getting an adequate number of nutrients and minerals in your day-to-day diet while pregnant. You ought to take a pre-birth nutrient enhancement to ensure you are reliably getting an adequate number of nutrients and minerals consistently. Your primary care physician can suggest an over-the-counter brand or recommend a pre-birth nutrient for you.

Eat and drink no less than four servings of dairy items and calcium-rich food sources a day to assist with guaranteeing that you are getting 1,000-1,300 milligrams (mg) of calcium in your day-to-day diet during pregnancy.

Eat no less than three servings of iron-rich food sources, like lean meats, spinach, beans, and breakfast grains every day to guarantee you are getting 27 milligrams (mg) of iron day to day.

While you're pregnant, you will require 220 micrograms (mcg) of iodine daily to assist with guaranteeing your child's mind and sensory system advancement. Try not to get exceeding 1,100 mcg daily. Browse an assortment of dairy items - - milk, cheddar (particularly curds), yogurt - - as well as heated potatoes, cooked naval force beans, and restricted sums - - 8 to 12 ounces (0.45 kg) each week - - of fish like cod, salmon, and shrimp.

Pick somewhere around one great wellspring of L-ascorbic acid consistently, for example, oranges, grapefruits, strawberries, honeydew, papaya, broccoli, cauliflower, Brussels fledglings, green or red peppers, tomatoes, and mustard greens. It makes it simpler for your body to assimilate iron from plant food varieties, constructs solid bones and teeth, supports susceptibility, and keeps areas of strength for veins red platelets sound. Pregnant ladies need

80-85 mg of L-ascorbic acid daily. Try not to surpass 2,000 mg.

Pick no less than one great wellspring of folate consistently, similar to dull green verdant vegetables, veal, and vegetables (Boma beans, dark beans, dark-looking peas and chickpeas). Each pregnant lady requires somewhere around 0.64 mg (around 600 mcg) of folate each day to assist with forestalling brain tube deformities, for example, spina bifida. Supplements called folic corrosive can be a significant choice when you are pregnant.

Pick no less than one wellspring of vitamin A and every other day. Wellsprings of vitamin An incorporate carrot, pumpkins, yams, spinach, water squash, turnip greens, beet greens, apricots, and melon.

Food varieties to Keep away from When Pregnant

Stay away from liquor during pregnancy. Liquor has been connected to unexpected labor, scholarly inability, birth deformities, and low birth weight children.

Limit caffeine to 300 mg each day. The caffeine content in different beverages relies upon the beans or leaves utilized, and the way things were ready. An 8-ounce mug of espresso has around 150 mg of caffeine on normal, while dark tea commonly has around 80 mg. A 12-ounce glass of stimulated soft drink contains somewhere in the range of 30-60 mg of caffeine. Keep in mind, chocolate (particularly dim chocolate) contains caffeine - - at times a giant sum.

The utilization of saccharin is unequivocally deterred during pregnancy, since it can cross the placenta and may stay in fetal tissues. In any case, the utilization of other non-nutritive or counterfeit sugars endorsed by the FDA is satisfactory during pregnancy. These FDA-supported sugars incorporate aspartame (Equivalent or NutraSweet), acesulfame-K (Sunset), and sucrose (Spend). These sugars are viewed as protected with some restraint, so speak with your medical services' supplier about how much non-nutritive sugar is adequate during pregnancy.

Decline the aggregate sum of fat you eat to 30% or less of your absolute everyday calories. For an individual eating 2000 calories every day, this would be 65 grams of fat or less each day.

Limit cholesterol admission to 300 mg or less each day.

Try not to eat shark, swordfish, cultivated salmon (wild is alright), ruler mackerel, or tile fish (likewise called white snapper), since they contain elevated degrees of mercury. An excessive amount of mercury can hurt your child's focal sensory system.

Keep away from delicate cheeses, for example, feta, Brie, Camembert, blue-veined, and Mexican-style cheddar. These cheeses are frequently unpasteurized and may cause Listeria disease. There's a compelling reason to keep away from hard cheddar, handled cheddar, cream cheddar, curds, or yogurt.

Stay away from crude fish, particularly shellfish like shellfish and mollusks.

What to Eat When Pregnant and Don't Feel Good

During pregnancy, you might have morning affliction, the runs, or blockage. You might find it hard to hold food varieties down, or you might feel excessively debilitated to try to eat by any means. Here are a few ideas:

Morning ailment:

Eat saltines, cereal, or pretzels before getting up; eat little, successive dinners over the course of the day; stay away from greasy, seared, fiery, and oily food varieties.

Blockage:

Eat all the new products of the soil. Likewise, drink 6 to 8 glasses of water a day. Taking fiber enhancements may likewise help. Check with your primary care physician first.

The runs:

Eat more food varieties that contain gelatin and gums (two kinds of dietary fiber) to assist with retaining abundance of water. Instances of these food sources are fruit purée, bananas, white rice, oats, and refined wheat bread.

Acid reflux:

Eat little, regular feasts over the course of the day; take a stab at drinking milk before eating; and break point jazzed food sources and refreshments, citrus refreshments, and fiery food sources.

Could I at any point eat fewer carbs While Pregnant

No. Try not to slim down or attempt to get thinner during pregnancy - - both you and your child need the appropriate supplements to be solid. Remember that you will lose some weight the main week your child is conceived.

Complex Sugars When Pregnant

For what reason Do I Want Complex Sugars While Pregnant?

Complex carbs give your body the energy it necessitates to make all the difference for you and develop all through your pregnancy. They're likewise loaded with fiber, which assists with processing and forestalling blockage, frequently a worry for pregnant ladies.

Complex carbs include:

Foods grown from the ground

Entire grains like oats, earthy colored rice, entire wheat breads, and pastas

Could I at any point eat a 'Low-Carb' Diet When Pregnant?

Low-starch slims down, for example, Atkins and the South Oceanside Eating routine, are exceptionally famous. There have been no investigations of the impacts of a low-carb diet on pregnancy, so its impact on the baby, if any, are obscure. While you are pregnant, you ought to eat a decent eating regimen, from all the nutritional categories.

Could I at any point Keep up with My Vegan Diet When Pregnant?

Since you are pregnant doesn't mean you need to wander from your veggie lover diet. Your child can get all the nourishment they need to develop and create while you follow a veggie lover diet, on the off chance that you ensure you eat a wide assortment of quality food sources that give sufficient protein and calories to you and your child.

Contingent upon the kind of vegan feast plan you follow, you might have to change your dietary patterns to guarantee that you and your child are getting satisfactory sustenance. Examine your eating regimen with your PCP.

Calcium When Pregnant

For what reason Do I Want More Calcium When Pregnant?

Calcium is a supplement required in the body to areas of strength for construction and bones. Calcium likewise permits blood to cluster typically, muscles and nerves to work appropriately, and the heart to ordinarily thump.

A large portion of the calcium in your body is tracked down inside your bones.

Your developing child needs a lot of calcium to create. If you don't consume sufficient calcium to support the requirements of your creating child, your body will take calcium from your bones, diminishing your bone mass and seriously jeopardizing you for osteoporosis. Osteoporosis causes emotional diminishing of the bone, bringing about powerless, fragile bones that can undoubtedly be broken.

Pregnancy is a crucial time for a lady to consume more calcium. It might assist with forestalling hypertension while you're pregnant. Regardless of whether no issues are created during pregnancy, a lacking stockpile of calcium as of now can reduce bone strength and increase your risk for osteoporosis sometime down the road.

The accompanying rules will assist with guaranteeing that you are consuming sufficient calcium all through your pregnancy:

The U.S. Suggested Day-to-day Stipend (RDA) for calcium is 1,000 mg each day for pregnant and breastfeeding ladies over age 18. The U.S. RDA for young ladies up to mature 18 is 1,300 mg of calcium each day. Try not to surpass 2,500 mg daily.
Eating and drinking no less than four servings of dairy items and calcium-rich food sources a day will assist with guaranteeing that you are getting the fitting measure of calcium in your day-to-day diet.

The best wellsprings of calcium are dairy items, including milk, cheddar, yogurt, cream soups, and pudding. Calcium is additionally found in food sources including green vegetables (broccoli, spinach, and greens), fish, dried peas, and beans. A few juices and tofu are made with calcium.

Vitamin D will assist your body with utilizing calcium. Go for the gold units (IU) a day however, something like 4,000 IU. You can help vitamin D through openness to the sun and in sustained milk, eggs, and fish.

How Might I Get Sufficient Calcium, assuming I'm Lactose Narrow minded?

Lactose narrow-mindedness is the failure to process lactose, the sugar tracked down in milk. On the off chance that you are lactose bigoted, you might have squeezing, gas, or looseness of the bowels when dairy items are consumed.

If you are lactose prejudiced, you can in any case get the calcium you really want. Here are a few ideas:

Use Lactate Milk braced with calcium. Converse with your dietitian about other lactose-diminished items.

You might have the option to endure specific milk items that contain less sugar, including cheddar, yogurt, and curds.

Eat non-dairy calcium sources, including greens, broccoli, sardines, and tofu.

Take a stab at drinking modest quantities of milk with dinners. Milk is better endured with food.

Would it be a good idea for me to take a Calcium Enhance During Pregnancy

On the off chance that you experience difficulty eating sufficient calcium-rich food sources in your everyday feast plan, converse with your PCP or dietitian about taking a calcium supplement. How much calcium you will require from an enhancement relies on how much calcium you are devouring through food sources.

Calcium enhancements and a few acid neutralizers containing calcium, like Tums, may supplement a generally solid eating regimen. Numerous nutrient enhancements contain next to zero calcium; in this way, you might require an extra calcium supplement.

Iron During Pregnancy

For what reason Do I Want More Iron During Pregnancy

Iron is a mineral that makes up a significant piece of hemoglobin, the substance in blood that conveys oxygen all through the body. Iron likewise conveys oxygen to muscles, assisting them with working appropriately. Iron aides increment your protection from stress and sickness.

The body assimilates iron all the more proficiently during pregnancy; hence, it is essential to consume more iron while you are pregnant to guarantee that you and your child are getting sufficient oxygen. Iron will likewise assist you with staying away from side effects of sluggishness, shortcoming, crabbiness, and sorrow.

Following a decent eating routine and incorporating food varieties high in iron can assist with guaranteeing that you are devouring sufficient iron all through your pregnancy. What's more, the accompanying rules will help:

The U.S. RDA for iron is 27 mg each day for pregnant ladies and 9-10 mg for breastfeeding ladies. Try not to surpass 45 mg daily.
Eating about three servings of iron-rich food varieties daily will assist with guaranteeing that you are getting 27 mg of iron in your day-to-day diet. One of the most incredible ways of getting iron from your eating routine is to consume a profoundly sustained breakfast cereal. Note that iron admission isn't equivalent to press retention.

Retention of iron into the body is most prominent with meat wellsprings of iron, like liver.

What Are Great Wellsprings of Iron?

Meat and fish: Lean hamburger, chicken, shellfishes, crab, egg yolk, fish, sheep, liver, clams, pork, sardines, shrimp, turkey, and veal

Vegetables: Dark looked at peas, broccoli, Brussels fledglings, collard and turnip greens, Boma beans, yams, and spinach

Vegetables: Dry beans and peas, lentils, and soybeans

Natural products: All berries, apricots, dried natural products, including prunes, raisins and apricots, grapes, grapefruit, oranges, plums, prune juice, and watermelon

Breads and cereals: Enhanced rice and pasta, delicate pretzel, and entire grain and advanced or sustained breads and cereals

Different food varieties: Molasses, peanuts, pine nuts, pumpkin, or squash seeds

Would it be a good idea for me to take an Iron Enhancement During Pregnancy?

Converse with your medical care supplier about an iron enhancement. The Public Foundation of Sciences suggests that all pregnant ladies following a decent eating routine take an iron enhancement giving 27 mg of iron during the second and third trimesters of pregnancy (that is the sum of most pre-birth nutrients). Your primary care physician might build this portion assuming that you become sickly. In lack of iron, weakness is a condition wherein the size and number of red platelets are diminished. This condition might result from deficient admission of iron or from blood misfortune.

Different Realities About Iron

L-ascorbic acid assists your body with utilizing iron. It is essential to incorporate wellsprings of L-ascorbic acid alongside food varieties containing endlessly iron enhancements.

Caffeine can hinder the ingestion of iron. Attempt to polish off iron enhancements and food varieties high in iron something like one to three hours prior or after drinking or eating food varieties containing caffeine.

Iron is lost in cooking a few food sources. To hold iron, cook food sources in a negligible measure of water and for the most limited conceivable time. Likewise, cooking in cast iron pots can add iron to food varieties.

Blockage is a typical result of taking iron enhancements. To assist with easing clogging, gradually increment the fiber in your eating regimen by including entire grain breads, cereals, organic products, and vegetables. Drinking no less than eight cups of liquids every day and expanding moderate activity (as suggested by your PCP) can likewise assist you with keeping away from stoppage.

Other Significant Supplements

Choline forestalls issues in your child's spinal line and mind, called brain tube deformities, and lifts mental health. It additionally upholds your bones and may assist with forestalling hypertension.

The RDA is 450 mg; don't go more than 3,500 mg daily.

Eggs are extraordinary wellsprings of choline; one cooked egg has 272 mg. You can find it in meats like chicken, hamburger, and pork and in fish like cod and salmon. Broccoli and cauliflower additionally have choline.

DHA

Docosahexaenoic corrosive (DHA) is one of the omega-3 unsaturated fats. It helps support your child's mental health and vision. It might likewise lessen your gamble of coronary illness.

The RDA is 300 mg.

DHA can be found in fish like salmon, crab, fish, and catfish. Strengthened eggs are likewise great sources.

Potassium

Potassium assists you with holding your circulatory strain under tight restraints and keeping a legitimate liquid equilibrium. It's likewise essential for an ordinary heartbeat and energy.

The RDA is 4,700 mg.

The best food sources to eat for potassium are white beans, winter squash, spinach, lentils, yam, squeezed orange, broccoli, melon, and raisins.

Riboflavin

Your body needs riboflavin (now and again known as vitamin B2) to make energy and utilize the protein from food. It might likewise assist with lessening the gamble of toxemia.

The RDA is 1.4 mg.

Search for riboflavin in food sources like some morning meal cereals, eggs, almonds, spinach, broccoli, chicken, salmon, hamburger, milk, yogurt, and curds.

Vitamin B6.

B6 assists your body with making protein for new cells, supports your resistant framework, and helps structure red platelets.

The RDA is 1.9 mg. Except if your PCP endorses vitamin B6, don't take exceeding 100 mg daily.

B6 can be found in some morning meal oats, garbanzo beans, prepared potatoes with skin, hamburger, chicken, pork, and halibut.

Vitamin B12.

B12 assists your body with making red platelets and utilizing fat and sugars for energy. It additionally forestalls megaloblastic paleness, which can cause you to feel frail and tired.

The RDA is 2.6 mcg.
B12 can be found in food sources like salmon, trout, fish, meat, and a few grains.
Zinc

Zinc supports your child's mental health. Your body likewise needs it to develop and fix cells and make energy.

The RDA is 11 mg; don't surpass 40 mg.
The best food hotspots for zinc are cooked shellfish, meat, crab, pork, white beans, and some morning meal grains.

Chapter 2:

Pregnancy Superfoods

Make the most of those additional calories with these supplement stuffed decisions:

Beans

Chickpeas, lentils, dark beans, and soybeans have fiber, protein, iron, folate, calcium, and zinc. Appreciate in stew and soups, mixed greens, and pasta dishes, or as hummus with entire grain saltines or in roll-up sandwiches.

Meat

Lean cuts, for example, top sirloin steak pack protein, nutrients B6 and B12, and niacin, as well as zinc and iron, in structures that are not difficult to retain. Hamburgers are likewise wealthy in choline. Add lean ground hamburger to pasta sauces, or use it in tacos, as burgers, in pan sear dishes, and in bean stew.

Berries

They're loaded with sugars, L-ascorbic acid, potassium, folate, fiber, and liquid. The phytonutrients in berries are normally helpful plant intensifiers that safeguard cells from harm. Appreciate them on top of the entire grain oat, in smoothies made with yogurt or milk, in hotcakes, and in servings of mixed greens. Layer yogurt with berries and crunchy entire grain cereal for a pastry parfait.

Broccoli

It has folate, fiber, calcium, lutein, zeaxanthin, and carotenoids for solid vision, and potassium for liquid equilibrium and typical circulatory strain. Broccoli likewise has the unrefined substances for your body to make vitamin A. Eat it as a feature of pasta and pan-fried food dishes, steamed and finished off with a hint of olive oil, puréed and added to soups, or cooked: hack broccoli into scaled down pieces, cover daintily with olive oil, and meal on a baking sheet at 400 degrees until delicate, around 15 minutes.

Cheddar (purified).

Cheddar has concentrated measures of calcium, phosphorus, and magnesium for your bones and your child's, in addition to vitamin B12 and protein. Utilize decreased fat assortments to save money on calories, fat, and cholesterol. Nibble on it with entire grain wafers or natural products, sprinkle it on top of soups, or use it in servings of mixed greens, sandwiches, and omelets.

Eggs

These are the highest quality level of protein, since they have every one of the amino acids you and your child need to flourish. They likewise incorporate exceeding twelve nutrients and minerals, like choline, lutein, and zeaxanthin. Certain brands supply the omega-3 fats a Child needs for mental health and pinnacle vision, so actually look at the mark. Appreciate them in omelets and frittatas; in servings of mixed greens and sandwiches; in handcrafted waffles, crêpes, and entire grain French toast; and as bites, hard-cooked or mixed.

Milk

It's an incredible wellspring of calcium, phosphorus, and vitamin D. Milk likewise packs protein, vitamin A, and B nutrients. Pick plain or seasoned, and use it in smoothies with natural product, over entire grain oat and natural product, and in pudding; make cereal in the microwave with milk rather than water.

Squeezed orange (invigorated)

Squeezed orange with added calcium and vitamin D has similar levels of these supplements as milk. In addition, you get robust portions of L-ascorbic acid, potassium, and folate. Appreciate it plain or frozen as pops or ice solid shapes, and in smoothies.

Pork Tenderloin

It's just about as inclined as boneless, skinless chicken bosom, and it presents the B nutrients thiamine and niacin, vitamin B6, zinc, iron, and choline. Attempt it barbecued, seared, or heated.

Salmon

Eat this for the protein, the B nutrients, and the omega-3 fats that advance mental health and vision in children. Appreciate it barbecued or seared, or utilize canned salmon in servings of mixed greens and sandwiches.

Yam

This packs L-ascorbic acid, folate, fiber, and carotenoids, which your body converts to vitamin A. It likewise supplies potassium in massive sums. Appreciate heated, cut chilly, cooked, or stripped potatoes for bites and side dishes; squashed with squeezed orange; and simmered: Cut washed yam into wedges, cover delicately with canola oil, and meal on a baking sheet at 400 degrees until delicate, around 15 to 20 minutes.

Entire Grains

Advanced entire grains are strengthened with folic corrosive and other B nutrients, iron, and zinc. Entire grains have more fiber and follow supplements than handled grains like white bread, white rice, and white flour. Have cereal for breakfast; entire grain breads for sandwiches; earthy colored rice, wild rice, entire wheat pasta, or quinoa for supper; and popcorn or entire grain saltines for snacks.

Yogurt (plain, low-fat or sans fat)

Yogurt is loaded with protein, calcium, B nutrients, and zinc. Plain yogurt has more calcium than milk. Mix in natural product jam or honey, new or dried natural product, or crunchy entire grain oat. Utilize plain yogurt to top cooked yams or to make smoothies.

Chapter 3:

Solid Food During Pregnancy

Solid Snacks During Pregnancy

As yet searching for a method for getting those additional calories? Bites can get the job done. Be that as it may, this doesn't mean a piece of candy or a pack of potato chips. All things being equal, stock up on cereal, nuts, organic products, and low-fat yogurt.

Adding those an additional 500 calories in a sound manner can be basically as straightforward as eating:

25 almonds, low-salt or unsalted (220 calories).
⅔ cup was dried cranberries (280 calories)

½ cup blended nuts, low—salt or unsalted (410 calories), and 1 enormous orange (90 calories)

1½ cups little pasta shells (290 calories) with 1 cup (0.24 liters) cherry tomatoes (30 calories), ⅓ cup dark beans (80 calories), 2 tsp olive oil (80 calories), and a sprinkle of vinegar

For a more modest nibble of around 300 to 350 calories, consider:

1½ cups oats (220 calories) with 7 massive strawberries (40 calories) and ½ cup blueberries (40 calories)

7 egg whites (120 calories) with 2 servings of salsa (40 calories) on 3 delicate corn tortillas (180 calories)

2 cups (0.47 liters) low-fat yogurt (280 calories) and 1 huge peach (60 calories)

Partaking in a sweet or pungent treat once in a while it is alright. However, do it with some restraint, very much as you did before you were pregnant. A lot of salt can cause you to hold water and raise your circulatory strain, which isn't really great for you or your child. What's more, such many sweet food varieties will top you off with void calories, so you're less ravenous for the nutritious food sources that you and your child need.

Food Desires During Pregnancy

Food desires during pregnancy are ordinary. Although there is not a great reason for food desires, close to 66% of all pregnant ladies have them. If you foster an unexpected desire for a specific food, feel free to enjoy your hankering on the off chance that it gives energy or a fundamental supplement. In any case, on the off chance that your hankering endures and keeps you from getting other fundamental supplements in your eating regimen, attempt to make to a greater degree an equilibrium in your day-to-day diet during pregnancy.

During pregnancy, your preference for specific food sources might change.

You may abruptly loathe food varieties you were partial to before you became pregnant. Moreover, during pregnancy, a few ladies feel compelling impulses to eat non-food things, for example, ice, clothing starch, soil, mud, chalk, remains, or paint chips. This is called pica, and it could be related to a lack of iron, like frailty. Try not to yield to these non-food desires - - they can be destructive to both you and your child. Tell your medical services' supplier, assuming you have these non-food desires.

Assuming you have any issues that keep you from eating adjusted feasts and putting on weight appropriately, ask your medical care supplier for exhortation. Enlisted dietitians - - the sustenance specialists - - are accessible to assist you with keeping up with great nourishment all through your pregnancy.

Which food varieties to eat and keep away from during pregnancy

Food sources to keep away from

Weight gain

Supplements

Synopsis

We incorporate items we believe are valuable for our pursuers. If you purchase through joins on this page, we might procure a little commission. Here is our cycle.

Having a sound eating routine is crucial during pregnancy. Ideal nourishment can assist an individual with fulfilling the expanded actual needs of pregnancy and assist the baby with creating.

For a solid pregnancy, an individual's eating regimen ought to incorporate an equilibrium of proteins, sugars, and fats.

Notwithstanding, a few food varieties and beverages, like liquor and a few cheeses, can unfavorably affect a pregnant individual's wellbeing and the possible strength of their child.

Rules and procedures

Mathieu Studio/Stocks

Clinical experts suggest having a fair eating routine wealthy in supplementing thick food sources, including different creature and plant-based proteins, organic products, grains, and vegetables during pregnancy.

They suggest focusing on the accompanying food sources:

Products of the soil

Presently, around 90%Trusted Wellspring of the US populace doesn't get the everyday proposed admission of vegetables. To adhere to the public rules, hold back nothing .5 cups (1.18 liters) of vegetables and 2 cups (0.47 liters) of organic product each day.

An individual can hit these objectives by polishing off an assortment of new, frozen, or canned produce and 100 percent natural product juices. Notwithstanding, if conceivable, decide on an entire, new or frozen natural product rather than juice.

Chapter 4:

Best Natural Products to eat during Pregnancy.

Complex starches

Complex sugars incorporate dull vegetables, for example, yams and butternut squash, entire grains, for example, Fargo and buckwheat, and vegetables, like beans or chickpeas.

Decide on these rather than refined starches, which are in white breads, pastas, and rice whenever the situation allows.

Likewise, pregnant individuals with high glucose might have to painstakingly screen their starch admission. An individual's clinical group, including their obstetrician-gynecologist and an enlisted dietitian, can assist with fostering an ideal sugar focus for every individual.

Complex carbs give energy and are a decent wellspring of fiber, which is significant during pregnancy.

Become familiar with what recognizes complex starches.

Protein

Pregnancy is a time of fast development and improvement. Subsequently, getting the ideal measure of protein is a critical Trusted Source.

During pregnancy, it is vital to zero in on a scope of protein sources as a component of a reasonable eating routine.

Coming up next are great plant-based wellsprings of protein:

Plant-based protein powders, for example, pea protein powders

tofu and soy items

beans, lentils, vegetables, nuts, seeds, and nut margarine

Become familiar with plant-based proteins here.

Creature-based protein, from chicken, fish, meat, or eggs, for instance, can likewise be a piece of a sound pregnancy diet, and these contain all fundamental amino acids.

Dive more deeply into the distinctions between plant-based and creature proteins here.

Fats are a vital part of the Trusted Wellspring of any solid eating routine and assume a critical part during pregnancy. Nonetheless, the sorts of fat are significant. For instance, getting omega-3 polyunsaturated unsaturated fats is basic during pregnancy.

Furthermore, high admissions of soaked fat can build the gamble of pregnancy difficulties.

An individual can securely consume a few soaked fats during pregnancy, however for ideal wellbeing, they ought to have unsaturated fats on a more regular basis.
Find out about the distinctions among soaked and unsaturated fats.

Instances of food varieties wealthy in polyunsaturated fats include:

Greasy fish, like salmon, herring, and trout
flaxseeds and sunflower seeds

pecans

Find more food sources wealthy in polyunsaturated fats here.

Fiber

Entire grain food varieties like oats, earthy colored rice, beans and lentils, organic products, and vegetables are rich in fiber. These food sources add to by and large destroy wellbeing and can assist with people feeling more full for longer.

Having an eating regimen high in fiber can likewise lessen the gamble of creating entanglements related with pregnancy, like hemorrhoids and obstruction.

Supplement needs during pregnancy

An individual requires more water-and fat-solvent nutrients during pregnancy and lactation. This incorporates folate, choline, and nutrients B12, A, and D, among others.

Specialists typically Trusted Source encourage individuals to take pre-birth supplements previously, during, and after pregnancy to keep up with sound supplement levels and back their bodies through post pregnancy recuperation.

Iron and pregnancy

Iron makes up a critical piece of hemoglobin. Hemoglobin is the oxygen-conveying color and principal protein in red platelets.

During pregnancy, how much blood in the body increases by practically 50%Trusted Source. To make the extra hemoglobin in this blood, the body needs more iron.

On the off chance that iron stores are deficient, a pregnant individual might foster frailty. This expands the gamble of:

Sluggishness, peevishness, and gloom

preterm conveyance

a low weight for the child

stillbirth

Likewise, on the off chance that sickness grows later in the pregnancy, there is a higher gamble of the individual losing blood when they conceive an offspring.

The accompanying food varieties are rich wellsprings of iron:

Lean meats'

poultry

salmon

vegetables

dim green vegetables

For more science-upheld assets on sustenance, visit our committed center point.

Food sources to keep away from

To assist with forestalling sicknesses and different entanglements during a pregnancy, stay away from:

Fish that contains mercury: Stay away from shark, swordfish, and marlin, or downplay the admission.

Uncooked or to some degree cooked meats: Pick completely cooked meats.

Uncooked shellfish: This is because of a gamble of bacterial or viral defilement, which can cause food contamination.

Crude eggs: Keep away from these and any food varieties that contain them.

Delicate, shape matured cheddar: Cheeses, for example, brie and Camembert convey a gamble of Listeria tainting. Listeria is a gathering of microscopic organisms that can cause possibly deadly contamination in pregnant individuals and their children.

Should pregnant individuals totally quit drinking liquor?

There is no known safe measure of liquor during pregnancy. It is safest Trusted Source to drink none by any means.

Liquor in the blood passes to the baby by the umbilical line, and a lot of openness to liquor can genuinely subvert the fetal turn of events. Likewise, there is a gamble that the child will foster a fetal liquor range disorder Trusted Source. This can bring about vision or hearing issues, issues with consideration, and low body weight, among different intricacies.

Should pregnant individuals stay away from caffeine

Consuming an excess of caffeine during pregnancy is related with an expanded gamble of unsuccessful labor, fetal improvement issues, and a low birth weight.

A caffeine consumption as low as 100-200 milligrams (mg)Trusted Source each day could adversely affect fetal turn of events.

Numerous food sources and beverages apart from espresso contain caffeine. Models incorporate a few soft drinks, caffeinated beverages, chocolate, and teas. Some cold and influenza cures additionally contain caffeine. A specialist, medical attendant, or drug specialist can give more direction about which meds are protected.

Weight gain

Putting on the perfect proportion of weight during pregnancy is an important Trusted Hotspot for the child's well-being. The best sum relies upon an individual's weight list (BMI). We give more data underneath.

Notwithstanding, these are just proposals. A specialist can give explicit focuses to every individual considering their wellbeing.

Suggested weight an individual expecting a solitary child ought to acquire. Proposed weight an individual expecting twins ought to acquire. Notice

Supplements

An individual necessities a more significant amount of practically all the water-and fat-solvent supplements during pregnancy. Thus, clinical experts recommend Trusted Source taking pre-birth supplements previously, during, and after a pregnancy to help wellbeing and recuperation.

A balanced pre-birth supplement contains every one of the vital supplements. These include Trusted Source, yet are not restricted to:

Folate
choline
vitamin B12
iron
vitamin D
vitamin A
magnesium

An individual can search for pre-birth supplements here.

Iron

A pregnant individual ought to be consuming 27 mg Trusted Wellspring of iron each day. The vast majority can't get enough from a solid eating routine. Be that as it may, enhancements can help.

Folate

As indicated by the World Wellbeing Association (WHO), an individual ought to consume 400 mcg (micrograms)Trusted Wellspring of folic corrosive each day up to the twelfth seven-day stretch of pregnancy.

Vitamin D

Concentrates on gauge that 18-84%Trusted Wellspring of pregnant individuals overall have a lack of vitamin D.

Current rules express that an individual requires 15 mistrusted sources, or 600 worldwide units (IU), of vitamin D every day during pregnancy.

Be that as it may, some wellbeing experts trust this objective to be excessively low.

A few specialists have found that pregnant individuals need more like 4,000 Entrusted Sources each day to keep up with ideal vitamin D levels. Individuals who are bosom or chest feeding require around 6,400 Entrusted Sources each day.

Zinc

Taking zinc supplements during pregnancy may marginally lessen the gamble of preterm birth. Getting 11-12 mistrusted Sources each day might be sufficient.

Choline is significant for the wellbeing of the pregnant individual and their child. Concentrates to show that most pregnant ladies in the U.S. try not to get the suggested 450 mg Trusted Wellspring of choline each day. Numerous pre-birth nutrients don't contain it, so getting enough from the eating routine, for example, from eggs and shitake mushrooms, is a crucialTrusted Source.

Vitamin A, or retinol, is fundamental for wellbeing during pregnancy, yet an excess of it can be harmful. During pregnancy, an individual ought to consume 750-770 mcg of retinol or retinol movement reciprocals (RAE).

Vitamin A happens in different structures. RAE estimates the overall measure of the nutrient in these different structures.

One RAE is commonly identical to:

1 mcg of retinol

12 mcg of beta-carotene from food

2 mcg of beta-carotene from supplements

3.33 IU of vitamin A

Omega-3s are critical Trusted Hotspot for natal turn of events and an individual's general wellbeing during pregnancy.

Expanding the admission of omega-3 polyunsaturated unsaturated fats during pregnancy might decrease the frequency of preterm birth. An individual can do this through their eating regimen or through supplements.

Outline

Pregnancy expands the actual requests on the body. An individual can fit their eating regimen to fulfill these needs and back the fetal turn of events.

A pregnancy sustenance plan ought to include:

The ideal protein consumption, from plant and creature sources, like fish, chicken, eggs, and lentils

fiber-rich starches, from sources like oats, yams, and organic product

solid fats, from sources like avocados, nuts, seeds, olive oil, and yogurt

Furthermore, a pre-birth supplement can assist with giving the fundamental supplements to pregnancy, bosom or chest feeding, and post pregnancy recuperation.

Medical services experts suggest restricting or totally keeping away from caffeine, liquor, and half-cooked meat and eggs during pregnancy.

Likewise, an individual's strict and moral convictions might shape what they eat during pregnancy. It is consistently smart to counsel a specialist while arranging a pregnancy diet.

Chapter 5:

Everyday LIFE

FOOD and RECIPES

The 18 Best Food sources for Infants and Little children

give your kid a wholesome lift by consolidating these superfoods into their eating regimen.

Child eating food in high seat

Infants don't eat much considering their little stomachs, so their weight control plans must contain numerous supplements. Look at this intensive superfood list for age-suitable things, ones that are open, sustaining, and sneak up suddenly.

What Are Superfoods

While the term is generally new, superfoods are not. They are food sources which offer the greatest health advantages for insignificant calories. Superfoods are additionally loaded with nutrients and plentiful in minerals and cell reinforcements.

When Can Children Eat Superfoods

As a rule, the things in this superfood list are suitable for children a half year and more established, while arranged by your baby's eating abilities. Certain things — like meat, organic products, and vegetable purées — might be presented bit by bit sooner than a half year if your child is prepared for them. Simply recall that strong food varieties of any sort ought not be presented before 4 months old enough.

Inquire whether you don't know when to present specific food sources or which food sources are best for your child.

Child's Most memorable Food sources: How to Present Solids

From the age of 1, strong food will supplant a large part of the milk in your child's eating routine. Have a go at presenting a more extensive assortment of food sources, introduced by, and urge your child to take care of himself.

Best Superfoods for Infants and Babies

These 18 things give your little one fundamental nutrients, supplements, and minerals. Integrate them into their eating regimen for ideal medical advantages.

Bananas

They are loaded with sugars for supported energy, as well as fiber to help a solid gastrointestinal system. They're a completely versatile child food, really their simple to-strip bundling. While serving bananas to small children, ensure they are ready and completely pounded. More seasoned infants can eat slashed bananas as finger food.

Yams

It gives potassium, L-ascorbic acid, fiber, and beta-carotene — a cell reinforcement that forestalls particular kinds of disease and mops up free extremists. Most children lean toward yams over different vegetables, considering their normally sweet taste. When cooked and pounded, yams make a smooth purée that is not difficult to eat, in any event, for children who are simply beginning to progress to strong food varieties.

Avocados

It has the most noteworthy protein content of any organic product, and they're wealthy in monounsaturated fat — the "upside" sort of fat that forestalls coronary illness. Ensure you just serve child ready avocados. Wash the outside, then, at that point, eliminate the strip and crush well.

Eggs whites give protein, while the yolks contain zinc and nutrients A, D, E, and B12. The yolk additionally has choline, which examination shows is vital for mental health. Generally, pediatricians have encouraged guardians to not serve eggs — particularly egg whites — until after the primary year due to the potential for unfavorably susceptible responses. In any case, that counsel has changed, and a few specialists accept that eggs ought to be deferred exclusively in families that have a past filled with sensitivities. Ask your primary care physician for more data.

Carrots

It has a lot of beta-carotene, a cell reinforcement that gives them their orange tone. Beta-carotene changes over into vitamin An and assumes a part in development and solid vision. Cooking carrots draws out their regular pleasantness, which makes them interesting to infants, who are brought into the world with an inclination for sweet flavors. While making carrots for your little one, ensure they are cooked until extremely delicate. Then purée them, or work well for cooked diced carrots.

Yogurt

It gives your child calcium, protein, and phosphorus, which are significant for sound bones and teeth. It likewise has probiotics, a sort of good microscopic organism that helps to process and supports the insusceptible framework. Children need fat in their weight control plans, so pick entire milk yogurt over low-fat or without fat assortments. Additionally, stay away from seasoned yogurts, which are high in sugar.

Cheddar

In addition to the fact that cheddar contains protein, it likewise brags calcium and solid portions of riboflavin (vitamin B2), which helps convert protein, fat, and sugars into energy. Swiss cheddar specifically has a somewhat sweet taste that is requested by infants. Since cheddar can be a stifling risk, cut it into little, diced pieces.

Child cereal

Iron-invigorated newborn child oats give your child the iron they require for legitimate development and improvement. Infants are brought into the world with a stock of iron; however, it begins to run out around 5 to a half year. On the off chance that your child is simply beginning to eat solids, specialists suggest iron-braced rice oats as their most memorable food, since it's doubtful that different grains cause a hypersensitive response.

Chicken

is loaded with protein and vitamin B6, which is utilized to assist the body with separating energy from food. Infants should begin consistently eating food varieties containing sufficient measures of protein to help their quick development. If your child could do without the flavor of chicken all alone, blend it in with their number one natural product or vegetable.

Red meat gives a handily retained type of iron, which assists red platelets with conveying oxygen to cells and helps mental health. More youthful infants can have meat purées, while more seasoned children who can bite can have very much cooked, finely diced meat.

Butternut squash

Infants love the sweet taste of butternut squash — and it brags solid portions of the cell reinforcement beta-carotene, L-ascorbic acid, potassium, fiber, folate, B-nutrients, and, surprisingly, some omega-3 unsaturated fats. Basically, steam or bubble butternut squash until delicate, then purée until smooth.

Fish

Greasy fish like salmon swarms with fat-dissolvable nutrients and fundamental fats that help mental health, eye wellbeing, and the safe framework. What's more, white fish like haddock and cod give a truly necessary protein help? Fish can cause an unfavorably susceptible response, however, so converse with your pediatrician before acquainting it with your child.

Tomatoes are a wonderful wellspring of lycopene, a cell reinforcement shade that assists with forestalling malignant growth and coronary illness. Notwithstanding, research demonstrates the way that lycopene in tomatoes can be retained all the more effectively by the body, assuming the tomatoes have been cooked with just enough oil.

Peas

They are overflowing with vitamin K, a supplement that works close to calcium to fabricate sound bones. They likewise have cell reinforcement nutrients An and C, as well as folic corrosive, fiber, and B nutrients.

Broccoli

This is a genuine superfood for infants, because of high measures of L-ascorbic acid, beta-carotene, folic corrosive, iron, potassium, and fiber. Bubbling broccoli in water slices its

L-ascorbic acid substance down the middle, so it's ideal to steam or microwave it. On the off chance that your child isn't excited about the flavor of broccoli, blend it in with a sweet-tasting vegetable, for example, yam or butternut squash.

Pasta

is a decent wellspring of intricate starches, which furnish us with supported energy. For this reason, it's so famous with competitors. Take a stab at blending some entire grain pasta in with normal pasta to build the fiber content of the feast. Try to pick little shapes and cook until exceptionally delicate.

Raspberries

contain pelagic cohesiveness, which can assist with safeguarding us against malignant growth.

Of the relative multitude of natural products, raspberries pack the most fiber into the least calories.

Earthy colored rice

Earthy colored rice gives energy, some protein, B nutrients, and minerals. It's considerably more nutritious than white rice, since the last option loses a large portion of its significant minerals and nutrients during handling. The starch in rice is consumed gradually, subsequently giving a consistent arrival of glucose for supported energy.

Chapter 6:

Practice during Pregnancy

Central issues

At your most memorable pre-birth care exam, ask your medical services' supplier assuming activity during pregnancy is alright for you.

Sound pregnant ladies need no less than 2½ long stretches of oxygen consuming movement, such as strolling or swimming, every week.

Customary active work can assist with decreasing your gamble of pregnancy complexities and simplicity pregnancy distresses, similar to back torment.

A few exercises, similar to b-ball, hot yoga, downhill skiing, horseback riding and scuba plunging, aren't protected during pregnancy.

Is it protected to practice during pregnancy?

Converse with your medical services' supplier about practicing during pregnancy.

For most pregnant ladies, practicing is protected and smart for yourself as well as your child. Get some information about what sorts of exercises are protected during your pregnancy.

If you and your pregnancy are sound, practice won't build your gamble of having an unsuccessful labor (when a child bites the dust in the belly before 20 weeks of pregnancy), an untimely child (brought into the world before 37 weeks of pregnancy) or a child brought into the world with low birth weight (under 5 pounds (2.27 kg), 8 ounces (0.3 kg)).

Activity during pregnancy

Solid pregnant ladies need no less than 2½ long periods of moderate-force oxygen consuming action every week. Vigorous exercises cause you to inhale quicker and profoundly, and make your heart beat quicker. Moderate-force implies you're sufficiently dynamic to perspire and expand your pulse. Going for a lively stroll is an illustration of moderate-power, high-impact action. If you can't talk ordinarily during a movement, you might be really buckling down.

You don't need to do all 2½ hours without a moment's delay. All things considered, split it up as the week progressed. For instance, complete 30 minutes of activity on most or throughout the days. On the off chance that this sounds like a ton, split up the 30 minutes by accomplishing something dynamic for 10 minutes multiple times every day.

Why is dynamic work during pregnancy extraordinary for you

For strong pregnant women, typical movement can:

Keep your mind and body strong. Genuine work can assist you with feeling quite a bit improved and give you extra energy. It also makes your heart, lungs, and veins strong and helps you with staying fit.

Help you with putting on the ideal extent of weight during pregnancy

Work with a couple of typical upsets of pregnancy, like deterrent, back desolation and growing in your legs, lower legs and feet

help you with administering strain and rest better. Stress will be pressure, strain or pressure that you feel considering things that happen in your life.

Help with decreasing your risk of pregnancy traps, such as gestational diabetes and pre-eclampsia. Gestational diabetes is a kind that can happen during pregnancy. It happens when your body has an unnecessary measure of sugar (called glucose) in the blood. Pre-eclampsia is a sort of hypertension a couple of women get after the 20th multi day stretch of pregnancy or ensuing to imagine a posterity. These conditions can extend your bet of experiencing issues during pregnancy, such as unfavorable birth (birth before 37 weeks of pregnancy).

Help with decreasing your bet of having a cesarean birth (moreover called c-portion). Cesarean birth is an operation wherein your kid is brought into the world through a cut that your PCP makes in your stomach and uterus.

Set up your body for work and birth. Works out, for instance, pre-birth yoga and Pilates can help you with chipping away at breathing, reflection and other calming procedures that may be valuable to your direct work torture. Ordinary action can help with giving you energy and fortitude to navigate work.

What kinds of activities are safeguarded during pregnancy

Accepting at least for a moment that you're sound, and you rehearsed before you got pregnant, continuing with your activities during pregnancy is by and large safeguarded. Check with your provider, no question. For example, if you're a runner or a tennis player, or you do various kinds of phenomenal movements, you could have the choice to keep on doing your activities when you're pregnant. As your belly gets more noteworthy later in pregnancy, you could need to change a couple of activities or straightforwardness up on your activities.

Expecting your provider says it's Satisfactory for you to work out, pick practices you appreciate. If you didn't rehearse before you were pregnant, right now is an unprecedented chance to start. Chat with your provider about safe activities. Start slowly and foster your well-being continuously. For example, start with 5 minutes of activity consistently, and move step by step up to 30 minutes consistently.

Is active work alright for every pregnant lady

No. For certain ladies, practice isn't protected during pregnancy. Your supplier can assist you with understanding on the off chance that exercise is alright for you. The accompanying circumstances might make it risky to practice during pregnancy. Preterm work, draining from the vagina, or your water breaks (additionally called burst films). Preterm work is work that occurs before 37 weeks of pregnancy. Draining from the vagina and having your water break might be indications of preterm work.

Being pregnant with twins, trios or more (likewise called products) with other gamble factors for preterm work. Assuming you're pregnant with products, inquire whether it's safe for you to work out. Your supplier might ask you to avoid extraordinary or high-influence exercises, such as running. Be that as it may, you might have the option to do low-affect exercises, such as strolling, pre-birth yoga or swimming.

Cervical inadequacy or a declared. The cervix is the opening to the uterus (belly) that sits at the highest point of the vagina. Cervical deficiency (likewise called inept cervix) implies your cervix opens (expands) too soon during pregnancy, typically without torment or constrictions. Cervical inadequacy can cause untimely birth and premature delivery. If you have cervical deficiency or a short cervix, your supplier might suggest a circle. This is a line your supplier places in your cervix to assist with keeping it shut, so your child isn't conceived too soon. A short cervix implies the length of your cervix (likewise called cervical length) is more limited than ordinary.

Gestational hypertension or toxemia. Gestational hypertension is hypertension during pregnancy. It begins following 20 weeks of pregnancy and disappears after you conceive an offspring.

Placenta prefix following 26 weeks of pregnancy. This is the point at which the placenta lies extremely low in the uterus and covers all or part of the cervix. The placenta fills in your uterus and supplies the child with food and oxygen through the umbilical string. Placenta previa can cause weighty draining and different difficulties later in pregnancy.

Extreme paleness or certain heart or lung conditions. Weakness is the point at which you need more solid red platelets to convey oxygen to the remainder of your body. On the off chance that you show some care or lung condition, inquire whether it's protected to practice during pregnancy.

Exercises normally are protected during pregnancy

Strolling.

Going for an energetic stroll is an extraordinary exercise that doesn't strain your joints and muscles. On the off chance that you're new to work out, this is an incredible movement to begin with.

Swimming and water exercises.

The water upholds the heaviness of your developing child, and moving against it assists keep your heart with rating up. It's additionally kind to your joints and muscles. Assuming that you have low back torment when you do different exercises, take a stab at swimming.

Riding an exercise bike.

This is more secure than riding an ordinary bike during pregnancy. You're less inclined to tumble off an exercise bike than an ordinary bicycle, even as your midsection develops.

Yoga and Pilates classes.

Tell your yoga or Pilates instructor that you're pregnant. The educator can help you later or keep away from representations that might be perilous for pregnant ladies, such as lying on your stomach or level on your back (after the primary trimester). A few rec centers and public venues offer pre-birth yoga and Pilates classes only for pregnant ladies.

Low-influence heart stimulating exercise classes During low-influence vigorous exercise, you generally have one foot on the ground or gear. . Instances of low-influence high-impact exercise incorporate strolling, riding an exercise bike and utilizing a curved machine. Low-influence vigorous exercise doesn't overwhelm your body that high-influence heart stimulating exercise does. During high-influence vigorous exercise, the two feet leave the ground simultaneously. Models incorporate running, working out with rope and doing bouncing jacks. Let your teacher know that you're pregnant, so they can assist you with adjusting your exercise, if necessary.

Strength preparing. Strength preparing can assist you with building muscle and making your bones solid. It's protected to work out with loads for however long they're not excessively weighty. Get some information about the amount you can lift.

You don't have to have a place with a rec center or own exceptional gear to be dynamic. You can stroll in a protected region or do practice recordings at home. Or on the other hand, observe ways of being dynamic in your regular daily existence, such as accomplishing yard work or using the stairwell rather than the lift.

What sorts of exercises aren't protected during Pregnancy

Be cautious and check with your supplier while picking your exercises. During pregnancy, don't do:

Any action that has a great deal of jerky, bobbing developments that might make you fall, similar to horseback riding, downhill skiing, rough terrain cycling, vaulting or skating.

Any game where you can get hit in the stomach, similar to ice hockey, boxing, soccer or ball.

Any activity that makes you lie level on your back (after the third month of pregnancy), like sit-ups. At the point when you lie on your back, your uterus comes down on a vein that carries blood to your heart. Lying on your back can cause your pulse to drop and restrict the progression of blood to your child.

Exercises that can make you hit water with incredible power, similar to water-skiing, surfing, or plunging.

Skydiving or scuba jumping. Scuba jumping can prompt decompression disorder. This is when risky gas bubbles structure in your child's body.

Practicing at high height (exceeding 6,000 feet (1.83 kilometers)), except if you inhabit a high elevation. Elevation is the level of something over the ground. For instance, assuming you're at high height, you're presumably in the mountains. Practicing at high heights during pregnancy can bring down how much oxygen that arrives at your child.

Exercises that might make your internal heat level too high, such as Bikram yoga (likewise called hot yoga) or practicing outside on hot, muggy days. During Bikram yoga, you do yoga in a room where the temperature is set to 95 F to 100 F. It's undependable for pregnant ladies since it can cause hyperthermia, a condition that happens when your internal heat level gets excessively high. A few examinations propose that investing a lot of energy in a sauna or hot tub might make your internal heat level excessively high and increase your gamble of having a child with birth. To be protected, don't spend over 15 minutes all at once in a sauna or more than 10 all at once minutes in a hot tub.

Pregnancy change how your body answers work out

During pregnancy, your body changes in numerous ways. At the point when you're dynamic, you might see changes in your:

Balance.

You might see that you lose your equilibrium all the more effectively during pregnancy.

Internal heat level. Your internal heat level is marginally higher during pregnancy, so you begin perspiring sooner than you did before pregnancy.

Relaxing.

As your child creates and your body transforms, you really want more oxygen. Your developing tummy comes down on your stomach, a muscle that assists you with relaxing. You might try to discover yourself feeling winded occasionally.

Energy.

Your body's striving to deal with your child, so you might have less energy during pregnancy.
Pulse. Your heart works harder and pulsates quicker during pregnancy to get oxygen to your child.

Joints.

Your body makes a higher amount of certain chemicals during pregnancy. This can make the tissues that help your joints more loose. Attempt to stay away from any developments that might strain or damage your joints. Chemicals will be synthetic compounds made by the body.
When would it be advisable for you to stop exercising? What are the admonition signs you ought to look for while working out?

While you're doing active work, hydrate and focus on your body and how you feel. Stop your movement and call your supplier, assuming you have any of these signs or side effects:

Draining from the vagina or liquid spilling from the vagina

Chest torment, quick heartbeat or inconvenience relaxing

feeling bleary-eyed or faint

Migraine

Muscle shortcoming, inconvenience strolling or torment or expanding in your lower legs. Torment or expanding in your lower legs might be indications of profound vein apoplexy (likewise called DVT). DVT happens when a blood coagulation structures in a vein somewhere down in the body, normally in the lower leg or thigh. On the off chance that, untreated, it can cause serious medical conditions and even demise.

Standard, difficult withdrawals. A withdrawal is the point at which the muscles of your uterus get tight and afterward unwind. Constrictions assist with pushing your child out of your uterus.

Your child quits moving. This might be a side effect of stillbirth (when a child bites the dust in the belly following 20 weeks of pregnancy.

When could you at any point begin practicing again after conceiving an offspring?

Converse with your wellbeing supplier to find out when it's Acceptable for you to be dynamic once more. On the off chance that you have a vaginal birth with practically no inconveniences, it's typically protected to begin practicing a couple of days after you conceive an offspring or when you're prepared. Vaginal birth is how most infants are conceived. During vaginal birth, the uterus agrees to assist with pushing your child out of the vagina (birth trench).

If you have a c-segment or a difficulty during birth, you might have to stand by longer to begin practicing after birth. Your supplier can assist you with deciding when your body is prepared to work out.

Assuming you were dynamic during pregnancy, it's more straightforward to get once again into practice after your child is conceived. Simply start gradually. Assuming you feel torment or have different issues during exercise, quit doing the action and converse with your supplier.

Chapter 7:

Stress and Pregnancy

Pressure Influence your Pregnancy

Feeling worried is normal during pregnancy, since pregnancy is a period of many changes. Your day-to-day life, your body, and your feelings are evolving. You might invite these changes; however, they can add new burdens to your life.

Elevated degrees of stress that go on for quite a while may cause medical issues, similar to hypertension and coronary illness. During pregnancy, stress can build in the possibilities of having an untimely child (brought into the world before 37 weeks of pregnancy) or a low-birthweight child (weighing under 5 pounds (2.27 kilogram), 8 ounces (0.3 kilogram)). Children conceived too early or too little are at expanded risk for medical issues.

Stress is a typical inclination during pregnancy. Actual distresses and different changes in your day-to-day existence can cause pressure during pregnancy.

A few sorts of pressure might cause serious medical conditions, similar to hypertension, and lead to issues like untimely birth.

Find out about ways of dealing with certain anxieties in your day-to-day existence like conversing with your medical services supplier and asking your accomplice, companions, or family for help.

How could post-horrible pressure issues influence pregnancy

Post-horrendous pressure issue (likewise called PTSD) is a problem that creates when you have issues after you experience a stunning, frightening or hazardous occasion. These occasions might incorporate assault, misuse, a cataclysmic event, a psychological oppressor assault or the passing of a friend or family member. Individuals with PTSD might have:

Serious tension

Flashbacks of the occasion

Bad dreams

Actual reactions (like a hustling heartbeat or perspiring) when helped to remember the occasion

Ladies who have PTSD might be more probable than ladies without it to have an untimely or low-birthweight baby. They likewise are more probable than different ladies to have hazardous wellbeing ways of behaving, for example, smoking cigarettes, drinking liquor, manhandling prescriptions or taking road drugs. Doing these things can expand the possibilities of having pregnancy issues. On the off chance that you figure you might have PTSD, converse with your supplier or an emotional well-being proficient. Medicines for PTSD incorporate prescriptions and treatment.

Could elevate degrees of stress in pregnancy influence your child's well being further down the road?

A few examinations indicate that elevated degrees of stress in pregnancy might create specific issues during youth, such as experiencing difficulty focusing or being afraid. It's conceivable that pressure likewise may influence your child's mental health or resistant framework.

Causes of Pressure during Pregnancy

The reasons for pressure are different for each lady, however here are a few normal causes during pregnancy:

You might be managing the inconveniences of pregnancy, such as morning disorder, clogging, being drained or having a spinal pain.

Your chemicals are changing, which can make your temperament change. Mind-set swings can make it harder to deal with pressure.

You might be stressed over what's in store during work and birth, or how to deal with your child.

If you work, you might need to oversee work undertakings and set up your group for when you take maternity leave.

You might stress over how you eat, drink and believe and what these things mean for your child.

What sorts of pressure can cause pregnancy issues?

Stress isn't all awful. At the point when you handle it right, a little pressure can assist you with taking on new difficulties. Normal pressure during pregnancy, like work cutoff times, presumably don't add to pregnancy issues.

Be that as it may, serious kinds of pressure during pregnancy might build your possibilities of specific issues, such as untimely birth. Most ladies who have serious pressure during pregnancy can have sound children. Be that as it may, converse with your medical care supplier on the off chance that you have these kinds of pressure:

Negative life altering situations. These are things like separation, difficult sickness or demise in the family, or losing an employment or home.

Devastating occasions. These incorporate seismic tremors, tropical storms or fearmonger assaults.

Enduring pressure.

This kind of pressure can be caused by generally disapproving of cash, being manhandled, being destitute or having serious medical conditions.

Wretchedness or tension. Wretchedness is an ailment that causes sensations of bitterness and a deficiency of interest in things you like to do. It can influence how you feel, think and act and can impede your day-to-day routine. It needs treatment to improve. Tension is a sensation of stress or feeling of dread toward things that might occur. The two circumstances might make it hard to deal with yourself and your child. Wretchedness and tension are normal and treatable, so converse with your supplier if you feel discouraged or restless. Assuming that you have these circumstances before pregnancy, converse with your supplier before halting or beginning any meds. Stopping out of nowhere can lead to difficult issues for yourself as well as your child. Assuming you want to quit taking medication or switch prescriptions, your medical services' supplier can assist you with making changes securely.

Neighborhood stress. A few ladies might have pressure from living in a neighborhood with destitution and wrongdoing.

Prejudice.

A few ladies might confront pressure from prejudice during their lives. This might assist with making sense of why African-American ladies in the US are bound to have untimely and low-birthweight children than ladies from other racial or ethnic gatherings.

How really does pressure cause pregnancy issues?

We don't totally figure out the impacts of weight on pregnancy. However, certain pressure related chemicals might assume a part in causing specific pregnancy difficulties. Serious or dependable pressure might influence your invulnerable framework, which shields you from disease. This can expand the possibilities of getting a disease of the uterus. This sort of disease can cause untimely birth.

Alternate ways stress can cause pregnancy issues include:

Ordinary pregnancy inconveniences, similar to inconvenience resting, body hurts, and morning disorder might feel far more atrocious with stress You might have issues eating, such as not eating enough or eating excessively. This can make you underweight or make you gain an excessive amount of weight during pregnancy. It likewise may build your gamble of having gestational diabetes and preterm work.

Stress might prompt hypertension during pregnancy. This jeopardizes you of a serious hypertension condition called toxemia, untimely birth and having a low-birthweight baby.

Stress additionally may influence how you answer specific circumstances. A few ladies manage pressure by smoking cigarettes, drinking liquor or taking road drugs, which can prompt serious medical issues in you and your child.

Numerous ladies stress that pressure might prompt premature delivery, the passing of a child before 20 weeks of pregnancy. While additional pressure isn't great for your general wellbeing, there's no proof that pressure causes premature delivery.

Pregnancy-related pressure.

A few ladies might feel serious fret over pregnancy. They might be stressed over pregnancy misfortune, the soundness of their child or about how they'll adapt to work and birth or becoming a parent. If you feel as such, converse with your medical services' supplier.

Decrease Pressure during pregnancy

Here are far to assist you with decreasing pressure:

Realize that the distresses of pregnancy are short-term. Get some information about how to deal with these distresses.

Remain solid and fit. Eat good food sources, get a lot of rest and exercise (with your supplier's alright). Exercise can assist with decreasing pressure and furthermore forestalls normal pregnancy inconveniences.

Scale back exercises you don't have to do. For instance, request that your accomplice assist with tasks around the house.

Attempt unwinding exercises, such as pre-birth yoga or reflection. They can assist you with overseeing pressure and get ready for work and birth.

Take a labor training class so you know what's in store during pregnancy and when your child shows up. Practice the breathing and unwinding strategies you learn in your group.

On the off chance that you're working, prepare to assist you and your boss with preparing for your time away from work. Utilize any time off you might need to get additional opportunity to unwind.

Individuals around you might assist with pressure alleviation as well. Here are far to diminish pressure with the assistance of others:

Have a decent encouraging group of people, which might incorporate your accomplice, loved ones. Or on the other hand, get some information about assets locally that might be useful.

Sort out what's making you focused and converse with your accomplice, a companion, family, or your supplier about it.

Assuming you figure you might have gloom or nervousness, converse with your supplier immediately. Seeking treatment early is significant for your wellbeing and your child's wellbeing.

Request help from individuals you trust. Acknowledge help when they offer. For instance, you might require help cleaning the house, or you might maintain that somebody should go with you to your pre-birth visits.

Chapter 8:

World Psychiatry

The World Mental Affiliation

Pre-birth psychological wellness and the impacts of weight on the baby and the kid. Should specialists look past mental issues?

Howard and Khalifa 1 give a careful outline of the scope of diagnosable mental problems that can happen in the perinatal period, along with their recurrence and techniques for treatment. They examine this regarding help both for the mother and to forestall conceivable antagonistic impacts on the kid.

Be that as it may, specialists and different experts might have the option to help regardless of whether the pregnant lady has a psychological issue. The proof recommends that there can be an expanded gamble to the future kid, assuming the mother feels worried, or has encountered early injury. It means a lot to think and help past determination.

A few unique sorts of pre-birth pressure for the mother have been displayed to expand the gamble of close to home, conduct and mental issues for the kid, and to assume a causal part. Such pressure in the mother incorporates her stress over the result of her pregnancy, her openness to a raised degree of day to day issues, to a characteristic or man-made debacle, and to close to home remorselessness or different types of homegrown maltreatment by her accomplice 2.

Outside stressors and the moms' levels of uneasiness and misery are many times much higher in low and center pay nations. In these nations, there can be extra pressure because of neediness, outside circumstances like conflict, more elevated levels of relational brutality, and explanations behind stress over the pregnancy result due to high newborn child or maternal mortality 3.

Assuming the mother is focused on during pregnancy, the kid is at an expanded hazard of side effects of nervousness and sadness, attention-deficit/hyperactivity jumble, lead jumble, and of being on the mentally unbalanced range. There can be different issues, including asthma and preterm conveyance. Severe pressure in the main trimester, like the passing of a more seasoned youngster or openness to a tremor, builds the gamble of later schizophrenia 4. With different results, there can be impacts all through pregnancy.

With this large number of impacts of pre-birth pressure, the proof shows that there is just an expansion in hazard to the future kid. Most youngsters are not impacted, and in the people who are, the level of the effect is variable. The individual hereditary weaknesses of the kid, and the idea of the post pregnancy care can likewise impact the result.

Youth abuse of the mother has been viewed as related with adjusted cerebrum structure in the infant, with decreased cortical dim matter. This affiliation was free of the mother's pre-birth temperament, and of other potential bewildering factors 5. This recommends that such early injury might influence the mother's science such that it modifies the advancement of the cerebrum of her hatchling, and may show weakness to later melancholy and different issues for the child.

The pathways by which these different kinds of pressure influence the lady's science, thus adjusting fetal neurodevelopmental, are not completely known. Be that as it may, a few pathways are being uncovered 6. These especially include the hypothalamic-pituitary-adrenal (HPA) pivot, and the insusceptible framework 7. The HPA pivot and other natural frameworks answer many outside stressors, and their reaction isn't related with explicit findings of dysfunctional behavior. There is proof that maternal and fetal cortisol levels are corresponded, particularly in additional restless or discouraged moms. On the off chance that the mother is restless or discouraged, this can change the capability of the placenta in a manner that permits more cortisol to go through to the hatchling. Raised maternal cortisol is related with modified cerebrum capability in the kid, remembering higher assimilating side effects for young ladies through modifications in neonatal amygdala network 8. Conceivable intervening elements for the impacts of early injury are those related with the resistant framework and aggravation.

If we can mediate to assist with diminishing burdens for pregnant ladies, we might have the option to forestall some kid neurodevelopmental issues. Therapists are prepared to analyze mental problems, and analysis is surely significant for treatment determination and anticipation. In any case, in certain settings it is critical to think past terms of explicit findings, and stress in pregnancy is one of them.

There have been endeavors to think in another manner about mental medical affliction. One is the advancement of the Exploration Space Models. This recommends another structure to give observationally based speculations about mental components that might be designated in mediations. This approach would be great if we had a natural test showing which pregnant ladies are probably going to be impacted in a manner connected to hurting the embryo and later youngster. We don't yet have such a test. We have close to zero familiarity with which organic changes in the mother intercede the consequences for the embryo.

In any case, we might in any case have the option to help. During pregnancy, practically all ladies have contact with wellbeing experts, who play a significant part in aiding both the lady and her future youngster. Wellbeing frameworks in various nations differ. However, specialists can assist with setting the plan. Many various kinds of pressure should be identified and tended to. This is an issue that ladies themselves see as significant. In a new survey, ladies picked "stress in pregnancy" as the subject most requiring expanded consideration from scientists, above others like sustenance or baby connection, corresponding to youngster improvement 9, albeit the creators of this study really do caution about the gamble of disturbing pregnant ladies about gentle to direct pressure.

In this way, it could be suitable for wellbeing experts really focusing on pregnant ladies to investigate parts of their psychological wellbeing which might be a wellspring of stress. How is the relationship with the accomplice? Did they experience the ill effects of early maltreatment or other unfavorable youth encounters? Do they have explicit tension about the result of their pregnancy? Have they been presented to some other significant anxieties, like fire or flood, or serious issues with cash or lodging? These are not questions generally investigated and may not prompt a particular finding. Yet, in dealing with pregnant ladies and in forestalling unfriendly results for their youngsters, we might have to think in new ways about emotional wellness in pregnancy.

We likewise may have to offer other help notwithstanding medications and talking treatments. These may incorporate assistance with the relationship with the accomplice. The dad is often a significant wellspring of stress, however can likewise be a significant help. This might include helping with viable issues like lodging, or working with the arrangement of a more grounded or more steady informal community.

The job of specialists and every one of those caring for the close to home wellbeing of women in the perinatal period, and for the future kid, is considerably more than assisting with analyzed mental problems.

www.ingramcontent.com/pod-product-compliance
Lightning Source LLC
LaVergne TN
LVHW010609160826
845677LV00013B/3318